Nothing But the Tooth

11 Questions You *Should* Ask Your Dentist

Stephanie Aldrich DDS FAGD FICOI

ISBN-10:1543189113
ISBN-13: 978-1543189117

DEDICATION

To my chosen family- Steven and Noah for being my strength and my chaos on a daily basis. I love you and your "male" ways!

To my loving parents- Frank and Debbie and sister- Heather- you've given me nothing less than encouragement and love. Thank ya and love ya!

To my Chi sisters- Amanda, Lara, Deanna, Corri, and Sarah- we've known each other for many years. It's been fun celebrating life with you! Cheers!

To my past, present, and future patients- thank you for trusting me with your health and allowing me to help make your smile one of your best features!

And finally to my wonderful kick-butt staff- Della, Kim, Leslie, Katie, and Brittany. Thanks for working hard and helping so many people! You're the best!

STEPHANIE ALDRICH DDS FAGD FICOI

CONTENTS

INTRODUCTION

So why am I writing this book? I am a pretty busy lady- I have a son who's starting school this year. I have a husband who is also a small business owner and works all the time. I am also active in martial arts and have many friends that I love to hang out with. And I also have a solo general dental practice where I see 40 patients a day, do all my own marketing, bookwork, and keep 5 staff members happy. And did I mention, I am studying for my Masters in General Dentistry? So why a book on dentistry?

Well, being in practice since 1999 and owning my own practice since 2000, I've seen a lot of mouths. I've seen a lot of things come in my practice that maybe wasn't handled the best way by other dentists. I've heard things that patients have told me that they've read off the internet or heard on TV and sometimes they are highly misinformed. And what am I supposed to say to these people? You're an idiot for believing these things?

Of course not!

However, after going to school for 20 years of my life, going through two fellowship programs on my way to my masters, and practicing since 1999, I feel like I am a little more educated on this subject and the questions that are in this book than let's say Wikipedia. So I thought this book may debunk some of the rumors that are out there and the he-said, she-said myths that go along with these dental subjects.

Some dentists and patients communicate differently and even though I'm sure my colleagues consult their patients on all of these things, it seems like the questions in this book cover themes that I tend to address over and over and over again. Every day I answer at least one of these questions.

Most are just plain common sense. But sometimes people have to hear it from an "authority" figure before they believe it. Well, let me be your authority figure. And if you don't believe me, go ask *your* dentist. Nothing I say in this book can be considered diagnostic per se, but it can help you ask your dentist the right questions and know that he/she is answering them for you completely and in a way that you understand.

Think of this book as a reference guide. Do you have a dry mouth and need something to help it, look in Chapter 9 about dry mouth symptoms. Do you have red puffy gums and want it to go away? Look in chapter 3 about puffy gums. I tried to not only tell you why something is occurring in your mouth, but what you can do to solve these issues. Then you can discuss this with your own dentist or specialist and know that they don't have to educate you on everything, they only have to look at your mouth and tell you what's the right choice of treatment for you, your mouth, and your budget.

Think of this book as your coach. I can't do these things for you, unless you live in Ohio or want to come visit me for your treatment- which of course I am happy to oblige! But I can guide you and educate you on your options so that nothing is missed and you're happy with the outcome of your treatment.

Most people that have problems with dentistry is usually because of fear of the unknown, or that there was a breakdown of communication between you the patient and the dentist. If you know what to expect, the cost, the time, the duration of the procedure, and the pros and cons of doing one procedure over another, usually you will have a satisfying outcome. But if any of the listed things are over-stepped or not discussed, then how can you be happy?

Most of the book discusses different situations that I see my patients in. I try to tell you what to expect, the time, the duration of the procedure, and the pros and cons of doing one procedure over another. The only thing I can't discuss in this book is the costs of procedures. This is because of insurance issues and also because of geography. Some insurances cover procedures and some don't. Some people have deductibles and some don't. Some people have to wait a year after receiving benefits while others can get something major done and have it covered right away.

Some parts of the country have different economics than other parts. A crown in Manhattan or LA will be a different price than a crown in Akron, Ohio simply because of local economics. But if I can give you some pointers on different procedures that your dentist can do, then all you have to do is discuss prices with them and which procedure is the best for you and your mouth. Then we can come up with a satisfactory plan of attack!

So use this book when you need it. If your grandma can't eat Christmas dinner because her dentures won't stay put, give her this book and have her read Chapter 8 on floppy dentures. If your nephew is 3 and still has a binky- give this book to your sister or sister-in-law and have her read Chapter 7. That's what I'm here for. The CSI agent on dentistry! Look at the facts and plan the case!

If you ever want to watch videos or keep up with my office schedule- go to www.akrondentalconcepts.com

Enjoy!

FORWARD

You're Never Fully Dressed Without A Smile
-Annie, The Broadway Musical

Trying to figure out what is best for you when it comes to dentistry can be overwhelming, time consuming, and flat out…frustrating. But with good information and an understanding of what your options are, that cloud of confusion can be cleared away and you can be freed up to make a decision that makes sense.

The connection between oral health and body health has been well documented in scientific literature. They call it this fancy terminology of "oral-systemic implications" which simply means teeth aren't separate from the rest of the body.

If something happens to them or there is disease in your mouth, it gets into the rest of body to put stress on organs like the heart, lungs, and brain causing a significant increased risk of heart attack and stroke. We have known that there is a link between gum disease and diabetes for years.

So we are at a time where teeth and your mouth aren't just about being able to smile with confidence and eat with comfort, they affect the quality of your life!

Dr. Charles Mayo, the famous physician for whom the world renowned medical clinic is named for, stated way back in the 1940's that a person's life span was reduced by 10 years just from not having healthy teeth!

I find that there is a huge gap between what you need as a patient and finding the right dentist for your dental care. We live in the information age, which on the surface should make it easier to get answers to your questions. But the truth is, the exact opposite occurs.

The shear amount of information, much of it weak or not applicable to your situation, bogs you down. And when you have to wade through that much content, your knee jerk reaction is to just quit.

So when I found out Dr. Stephanie Aldrich was putting together a simple-to-understand comprehensive guide for patients and their dental needs, I immediately thought, "Why didn't someone do this sooner?"

As someone who is also a licensed dentist, I see people who get in difficult situations that could have been avoided if they just knew a little more at the right time. Most dental problems can be resolved quicker, easier, and faster if they had just taken action a little sooner.

It's not your fault. You didn't know.

This book is to empower you! It gives you the straightforward, no nonsense basics that you need to help you on your oral (and total body!) decisions.

There are MANY options to prevent, repair, and replace your teeth. Advances are made every day to give people choices to have a healthy, attractive smile that they can keep for a lifetime with regular maintenance. That's why this resource guidebook is so valuable.

The reality is, most people give their cars more attention (and love) than they give to their own bodies. We would never think of missing 3 oil changes. Nor, would we ever substitute baby oil for the manufacturer's suggested motor oil, using the specified type and weight for your vehicle.

That would be totally insane! The results would be expensive auto repair bills and the loss of the use of our car. We couldn't function without it.

Your mouth deserves that same level of respect with regular maintenance and attention to repairs when they are minor to avoid bigger problems down the road.

In my own practice, I saw how someone's life could be completely changed with dentistry. Whether it was a 65 year old grandmother who could finally eat and smile because she now had a secure denture option that gave her back 90% of the function she had with her own natural teeth.

Or if it was like one of my favorite patients, a 7 year old boy who I met late Saturday night with an abscess the size of a golf ball because no one thought a big hole in his baby tooth would matter. His life changed because he was now completely pain free and had a healthy smile. He didn't have to miss anymore with his favorite soccer games.

Teeth matter.

As you go through this book, please remember you aren't reading this just for yourself. But for those you care about. Maybe it's your senior aged parents who have many health issues going on in their lives and need help when making decisions with their medical care. Or it could be a good friend that casually mentions he has a cracked tooth and he's going to put off going to the dentist because it "doesn't hurt right now".

With good information, there is power. And I hope you use this new knowledge to make your time more efficient.

Here's to your health,
Ginger Bratzel DDS.

CHAPTER 1

SHOULD I BE EATING NUTS AND CRUNCHY FOODS IF I HAVE A LOT OF DENTAL WORK IN MY MOUTH?

If I've learned anything about people's eating habits since I've been a dentist, it's that we as Americans love our crunchy foods. Whether it's kettle chips, sour dough pretzel nubs, wasabi peas, or almonds, we crave the crunch and the ability to use our muscle to crush these hard food items.

The only problem with this is that most Americans have some type of dental work done to their molar teeth- all of which are responsible for chewing our food.

Our genetic makeup says that because our back teeth are nice and flat, that we can be considered herbivores- eating nuts and plant-type food. But we also have 4 canines and sharper incisors in the front that can help to tear through meat. So we're really omnivores- eaters of everything!

So why is it that I am constantly repairing people's broken teeth and fillings? The easy answer is that people are eating too crunchy of foods. The more difficult answer is that the materials we as dentists are fixing the teeth with are causing more problems. So what is a crunchy-loving omnivore to do?

We as dentists only have a few materials to work with. Most of us try to pick the right material that is appropriate for the job. But not always. Some of us in the profession have biased opinions towards certain materials whether they are scientific opinions or otherwise.

I know for me, I try to use any or all materials that are available and try to use them in the best situations so that my patients get the longest duration of any restoration that I put in their mouth. But this is certainly a question to ask your dentist.

As I've said earlier, there are a few materials to work with. Amalgam, composite, porcelain, and gold. That's it. I'm hoping before I retire that we can introduce bone into the mix. HELLO! Teeth are bones!

Why can't we restore these teeth with bone? I know they're working on it, but it makes total sense to replace decayed bone with healthy bone- it has the exact same characteristics.

Porcelain and gold are used for crowns and bridge work. So to repair smaller holes in your teeth, we have amalgam (silver) fillings and plastic composite (bonded) fillings.

I personally use both for my patients. Large plastic composite bonded fillings don't last as long in molar teeth so I tend to either use sliver amalgam fillings for these teeth, or recommend to my patient to crown the tooth if they don't want the silver amalgam.

In a 2008 study in the Journal of Dental Research, Dr. Drummon studied two different ways that plastic composite bonded fillings fail. Years 0-5, the plastic composites tended to break.

In years 6-17, the fillings tended to leak causing cavities under the fillings. Also the plastic composite fillings have a compressive strength of 250mPa compared to amalgam's 414mPa. This basically means that amalgam is almost twice as strong as a composite filling.

So if you're a crunchy food person and have plastic composite bonded fillings in your mouth, you are very likely to either break the filling in the first 5 years, or cause the edges to leak, resulting in a cavity under the filling.

Most people like plastic composite bonded fillings for their look. They're tooth colored and tend to blend into the teeth. But I have many patients that love to chew ice, eat kettle chips and croutons.

I usually will recommend to these people either silver amalgam fillings or go one step further and put a porcelain crown on them.

At least with me giving you some options, you can make the best decision for your mouth. If you want composite fillings on your back teeth you can either give up the crunchy foods OR know that you're going to need to replace those fillings every 3-5 years.

The decision is always yours and your dentist should abide by your wishes. But don't hold him/her liable for a failing plastic composite filling that is only 2 years old when you're constantly crushing large chips against it. It simply won't last.

So the previous was about the fillings that you have and can break if you eat crunchy foods. But what about the actual tooth structure that's taking all the abuse? If the filling doesn't break, the other thing that could happen is that the tooth can break. Or start to fracture.

When there's a filling on the top part of the tooth where you chew, the filling itself can act like a wedge and start to split the tooth. It can cause small hairline fractures that start to spread throughout the enamel and possibly into the second part of the tooth called the dentin.

When the cracks start to occur, you may not feel anything. If you have a good dentist, the dentist will see these fracture lines and tell you about them. They may suggest that they can either watch these fracture lines because they don't bother you or that they remove these fracture lines and extend the filling to cover them.

If these fracture lines get worse, you can start feeling cold sensitivity, biting pressure, achiness, or a combination of all three. Usually if the fracture is on the surface- not through the enamel- you may only have biting pressure or no pain at all. If the fracture goes deeper, you may start to feel a combination of things.

If the cold or biting pressure or achiness is lingering and doesn't go away immediately after chewing food, the fracture may have gotten deep enough to affect the nerve. In this case, a root canal may be needed to clean out the nerve and bacteria that is festering in the tooth. This will help to relieve the pain.

So the question becomes- should you eat crunch foods if you have dental restorations in your mouth? In my opinion, no. I would lighten up on the crunchy stuff.

I'm not saying you have to eat baby food or blend up your food and drink it, I'm just saying that if you continue eating crunchy stuff, you are going to be visiting the dentist more often than you would probably like.

We also have to consider the point: how strong are your teeth to begin with? I can't tell you how many people I've seen over the years that simply have soft enamel.

When I do a filling on them, I have to be careful to just lightly touch their tooth structure because it's so soft to begin with. If you have a history of having a lot of fillings done you may be in this category.

Then my advice to you is: stop eating crunchy foods! Just don't even buy them. Unless you want to be spending a lot of time and money on your teeth.

Another consideration that I've discussed with my female patients is osteoporosis. After 35, females tend to have calcium and vitamin D problems, most of which can be attributed to child birth and the fact that we live in Ohio and get almost as much rain per year as Seattle.

Females should get their vitamin D levels checked. Vitamin D helps the body absorb calcium. Calcium is used to build bone. Teeth are bones.

Therefore we need both to help maintain our teeth. Over the years, I've actually helped to diagnose several patients with osteoporosis simply from the fact that they had awesome teeth and all of a sudden they started breaking them and having problems.

I've then pulled back from just being a dentist and suggested they do a blood work panel with their regular doctor to see if they indeed needed supplements.

The last tidbit of information that I will share with you is that I've also seen people come in with a split tooth and they don't even have any prior fillings on that tooth.

They are healthy and they ate something crunchy that caught their tooth in such a way to split it. Sometimes I can fix it either with a filling or a crown, but I've had other times that they have actually split the tooth in half and have required the tooth to be extracted.

So yeah, you can even split a tooth in half and end up losing the tooth - one that is healthy, just by eating crunchy foods.

So I hope this puts to rest my thoughts on crunchy foods. I only have one filling on a molar in my mouth and I don't eat crunchy stuff. I avoid almonds, kettle chips, croutons, and all hard candy.

I don't chew ice or popcorn kernels. There are two reasons why- the first is that I myself have that one filling on my molar because I ate a hard Cheetos and cracked the tooth. One that had never had a filling in there before.

The second reason is that I have made my living from you guys eating crunchy stuff and then expecting me to put you back together, which I'm happy to do.

But I warn everyone- eat crunchy foods at your own risk. If your dentist has not talked to you about your crunchy food habits and what types of fillings he/she should use, you need to have that talk.

If your dentist has not discussed how he/she has seen hairline fractures in your teeth that may need to be addressed soon, you need to have that talk.

Or if your dentist didn't give you the option of having a silver amalgam filling versus a plastic composite bonded filling because they just made that decision for you or they are a "cosmetic" dentist- a title that doesn't exist under the American Dental Association guidelines- and don't place silver amalgam fillings, then you still need to have that talk.

Or get another dentist. If you're in the Akron, Ohio area, give me a call. I'll give you all your options and we can come up with a longer-lasting solution to your crunchy habit!

And I know what you're thinking- "But I love my crunchy foods- I can't give those up!"

You can still eat your chips and almonds and croutons, but do me a favor. Don't eat them constantly every day. And look for alternatives. You can get chips that aren't salty bricks. You can get almonds that are sliced or slivered. You can eat croutons that aren't as hard as rocks.

Don't chew on ice cubes- get them crushed. As least they're not as hard and some will melt in your mouth before you have a chance to chomp on them. Look for alternatives!

CHAPTER 2

I DON'T HAVE DENTAL INSURANCE, HOW CAN I AFFORD THIS TREATMENT?

I think this question needs to be asked differently. If your dentist has recommended treatment, the real question is how can I *not* afford to get it done? I'm asked this question all of the time. I personally never ask, how can I afford it but rather how can I *not* afford it?

Something that you must consider when your dentist suggests a treatment procedure to you is, has he/she given you all of the treatment options, regardless of the costs, to you for your particular situation?

Being educated on your issue and what modern dentistry can do for you is the number one way to stay healthy throughout life. If you don't have a healthy mouth, you can't eat healthy foods and more than likely your overall health is poor. So getting all your options is the first thing to go over with your dentist.

The second thing to consider are the pros and cons of each of the treatment options that your dentist has laid out for you to consider. If you do procedure A, what are the pros of doing this now? Can I wait a few months to save up money?

If not, what is the timeframe that I am looking at to get this procedure done so that I have a successful outcome? What are the cons of picking procedure B over procedure A?

What are the long term ramifications of choosing this procedure over that one? Can I be hurting or affecting another part of my mouth if I choose this procedure over the other one? What are the success rates of having procedure A done compared to procedure B? Do you do more of procedure A than B?

By asking these types of questions, you can take the price issue off the table and really see what treatment you can live with and can meet your expectations.

For example- let's say you need a simple filling. It's going to cost $150. The tooth doesn't hurt and you decide to wait because life gets in the way and you'd rather spend that money somewhere else.

Over the course of the next year, you're eating something crunchy and suddenly you hear a 'crunch' and then that same tooth starts to hurt and it's hurting you so badly that it's keeping you up at night.

Now that tooth is way beyond a simple filling. Now the crack is probably in the nerve and now needs a root canal, a buildup, and a crown costing around $2000 or for $250 your dentist can yank the tooth out.

So something that could have been fixed with a simple filling can wind up costing you 10 times more because of a simple decision not to get it fixed now. I see this all the time.

That's why I always go over pros and cons with a patient and let them know what their choices are so that they can choose what their best course of treatment is, one that they can live with the consequences.

I just had a new patient come in with new dentures that were made by someone else. This poor lady couldn't even wear them because the other dentist didn't adjust them so they weren't hurting her.

She told me they weren't made right. After a little adjusting, she said they felt great! She noticed that the upper wouldn't stay in and I had suggested we reline the denture to help get her suction- she said her old dentist didn't say anything about relining them, that all he said was to use some paste.

I told her she still may need some paste, but usually a reline will help to fill in the gaps and help to create some suction. In one day, the lab did the reline and she now can talk and eat like she did when she had her own teeth.

She said she was so grateful that I told her the options she had and she acted on them. This is what I'm talking about. Too many people are in a rush and don't talk to their dentists about what's bothering them.

That's what we're here for! We're the CSI of dentistry. We try to figure out the problem and find a solution that is right for you and your situation. But it's all about communication! Ask questions. Nothing is dumb!

Make sure you know all the options before you make your decision. I never want one of my patients to tell me that they didn't know that this was an option.

No way! Not in my office!

I know that I can't be with everyone that's reading this book, but if I can be your big sister going in with you and arming you with some questions, I will certainly do that!

The third thing to consider is how you will feel about procedure A compared to procedure B. Some of my patients cannot fathom losing a tooth and will spend any amount of money and see any specialist in the area to keep their teeth.

Then I have other people that don't value their teeth at all and chuck them every chance that they get. More of these people are not in the best overall health and I assume they don't value their body in general, typically smoking and eating bad stuff and generally not living a healthy lifestyle.

Most of my patients fall in the middle. Most will want to be as conservative as possible but if they trust their dentist, will go along with whatever treatment their dentist recommends.

This brings up another thing to think about. Where is your dentist coming from? What's his/her style? Is he/she very conservative and middle-of-the-road or is he/she one of the elitist? If you have a problem with one of your teeth and your dentist is a conservative, he/she will probably either fill it or do other minor things to make it look good and make it feel better and function.

An elitist may want to totally pull the tooth and offer you a very expensive treatment plan just because they know they can without regards to what your opinion is. This is always something to think about when a treatment plan is given to you.

Do their opinions or style match up with your own? Are you a Type A personality that only wants the best? Or are you the type of person that's not highly concerned with your looks and not worried about whitening your teeth every 5 seconds or fixing that little chip that's on your front tooth?

Aligning your personal style with that of your dentist is very important to getting the treatment that you really want.

I always give my patients as many scenarios as I can possibly think of and then educate them on each with all of their pros and cons regardless of how much money it is.

I figure I am in the service business and it's my job to use my skills to make my patients happy AND functioning to the best of my ability.

But if you want to chuck teeth and your dentist only puts in implants, there will be a philosophical disconnect between you and him/her and you may want to find another dentist that has the same views as you do.

Another thing to consider is how long has your dentist been a dentist? Most dentists out of school less than 10 years don't have the longevity of their work to create a bias on what procedures and materials work and last in certain situations.

And then you have the older dentists that may not have had a continuing education course in decades. These people definitely aren't up on the latest technologies that can benefit their customers.

I think there's great dentists in every category, but you should be aware that not all are created equal. Look around their offices. Do they introduce different technologies and new procedures to their patients?

Do they need to reschedule your appointments once in a while because they are at a continuing education course? When you go in for a checkup, do they talk about courses or new procedures that they're doing now and telling you that you are a great candidate for it?

The last thing to consider is that if you don't have dental insurance, does your dentist offer payment plans? Sometimes they have companies like Care Credit that will help finance your procedure and then you can make payments like a credit card over a certain agreed upon term.

In my office, I have a discount fee plan that members can save 20-50%off our regular prices. We have been very successful in helping our patients remove the obstacle of money to help them achieve the smile that they want.

I personally have never let money dictate what I want or achieve. I grew up with a working dad and a stay-at-home mom. I paid for college with loans and some help from my parents. I started my practice all with loans at 11% interest.

It took me 13 years to pay off my $750,000 loan but I did it through a lot of sweat and a lot of hard work. There are so many ways to afford things. You can save the money by putting a little away with each paycheck.

You can arrange to have a little bit automatically taken out and put into a savings account so you don't even see it. You can ask a relative for the money. You can put it on a credit card. You can ask your bank for a loan.

You can use the money in your HSA account. You can borrow money out of your retirement account- only if you're going to pay it back of course. You can ask for financing from Care Credit or other dentistry-related places. If you know which treatment plan you want, you will find a way to pay for it.

You have a cell phone, don't you? A car? A house or apartment? Clothes on your back? Food in your belly? An IPad? An Xbox? Cable or satellite TV? Internet at home with Wi-Fi? Daycare? Etc. Etc.

 A lot of these things aren't necessarily things that you need, but they are things that you want and you've found ways to create the means to afford them. Think of your mouth and health the same way.

How can you afford *not* to fix it? To keep it healthy and strong. You will live a lot longer if you are able to eat healthy and not have constant infection, inflammation, and pain. Who wants that kind of life?

So don't look at it as *how* can I afford it? Look at it as how can I *not* afford to do it and then be creative and find the solution. If you need help, please give me a call and we can go through the treatment options and find one that fits your needs.

CHAPTER 3

MY GUMS ARE SO RED AND PUFFY- I COME TO THE DENTIST FOR MY REGULAR CHECKUPS- WHY?

This is a subject that no one teaches you in dental school. This comes from many years of seeing thousands of patients and being the CSI detective- asking the right questions and using deductive reasoning to find the solution.

There is one main culprit that explains an otherwise healthy mouth and red, sore, swollen gums. It's called whitening products.

If you look on the supermarket shelves, almost all oral health care products have some kind of whitening component in them. In the US alone, teeth whitening products amount to $1.4 billion! How white do we want our teeth?

Wow, that's a high number!

And it seems like more and more products contain some type of whitening component. It's such a fad right now and big companies are taking advantage of it. But at what price to the consumers?

The problem is, that most people don't know that the chief whitening component is peroxide and that peroxide is an acid. Over time, this acid eats away not only the organic stain that collects in the nooks and crannies of our teeth, but it also eats away at the soft tissue that it comes in contact with- like gums and cheeks causing major irritation and redness.

The peroxide breaks down into water and oxygen. It's the oxygen molecules that are very unstable and want to bind to something. They usually go after organic stains. But they can also go after other things like soft tissue- gums and cheeks, and also the nerve which can cause cold sensitivity.

Whitening products can also dehydrate the enamel, causing sensitivity. Anytime I do an in-office whitening procedure on one of my patients, I always tell them that if I see any chalkiness on their teeth, this is the beginning signs of the dehydration process and that we will stop the procedure because it will cause tooth sensitivity if we don't stop the procedure and that's not a fun thing to experience.

The PH of our products that we use in my office ranges from 3.5 to 5. If you remember from school, water has a PH of 7 so anything under 7 will have acidic affects.

Over-the-counter whitening products have a PH range of 5-11. Whitening toothpastes have a PH range of 4-6. So right away, most whitening products on the market are very acidic.

 The toothpastes seem to be the worst. And then you're using them 2-3 times a day, every day! No wonder people have problems!

Every day this acid is scrubbed into the gums and teeth and it takes time for the body's saliva and natural defenses to buffer this acid and return the mouth back to normal.

Then you drink your acidic coffee- PH of 5- and then you eat your salad full of tomatoes- PH of 4 and then you go home and use the toothpaste again- another PH of 4-6. And then you put on the whitening strips because your friends are doing it and all you're doing is causing havoc on your teeth and gums.

I have seen some horrible things walk into my office over the years. People that have healthy mouths come in with very red gums and say that it hurts and they can't even eat or drink without crying. It's terrible.

 I myself don't use any whitening products on a consistent basis. Even my own toothpaste is a plain gum defense toothpaste without whitening in it. I whiten my teeth every other year using my Zoom in-office whitening products.

That's it!

I don't carry strips around in my purse or use whitening swishes or toothpaste or coconut oil or anything like that. I use it when I build up stain and that's it. You're not going to build up stain in two seconds that's noticeable anyways, so why waste your money on that stuff? Don't get caught up in the commercialization of it or the fad of the times. It's just not that good for you and it's not a normal thing.

As dentists we have a shade guide that we use to try to match up the color of your teeth with restorative products like bonded white fillings and porcelain crowns.

There's only 16 shades on that shade guide plus a whitening shade. Everyone's teeth are different shades to begin with and then you put all the peroxide products on them and sometimes they become so white that there's no shade of product that will match.

This is definitely a problem if there's ever an accident and a front tooth is chipped. There's nothing on the market that will match it.

I've got one patient that is so obsessed with whitening her teeth that her teeth have a blueish tinge to them. I won't sell her any whitening products consistently. I always spread them out so I don't damage her enamel.

But she knows to be careful with her teeth because there's nothing out there that will match her color so if something breaks, she won't like the color of the restoration. So please be careful!

My best advice is to stop using any whitening product on a daily basis. If you want to do it once or twice a week, ok, but no more than that. That will help to break down any stain that has accumulated on the tooth surface but will not irritate the gum and cheek tissues.

Another culprit are acidic foods like tomatoes and strawberries. June is strawberry month in Ohio and August is tomato month.

During these times I will see people come in with red, sore, and swollen gums.

The first thing I will ask them is about the whitening products that we talked about earlier. The next thing I ask is if they're loading up on strawberries and/or tomatoes. Often they say yes! Then I tell them to calm it down, they're actually irritating their own gums for these acidic foods.

Another culprit is citrus fruits. Lemons, oranges, limes. I've seen kids come in who love to suck on lemons and usually their teeth have pits on the surfaces and their gums are very red and puffy.

Why?

Because lemon juice is very acidic and it's eating little holes in their teeth enamel and also irritating their gums. I usually will tell mom- stop it! Once in a while is ok, but don't give it to him/her every day, all day long!

Another culprit that can cause red swollen gums is spicy foods. This can be hot peppers, but it also can be synthetic cinnamon.

Cinnamon that comes naturally from the tree bark usually doesn't cause any problems, but hot cinnamon gums and candies can cause havoc on the mouth. I've seen large welts/blisters on people tongues from hot candies.

And it's not something that heals quickly either. In the summertime when everyone is making salsa- I will start seeing red swollen gums on patients.

Salsa is so good- I'm a Mexican food freak- you're getting the spiciness from the hot pepper oil, but then you're also getting the acid from the tomatoes- a double whammy! So make sure you're not eating salsa every day because it can cause problems.

For anything food related- the best way to calm things down is to stop eating these foods and rinse your mouth with warm salt water. This will kill the bacteria in your mouth and will have a healing, calming effect over the damaged tissues. The oils from spicy foods can also be neutralized with dairy products, that's a Mexican secret!

Another culprit to red puffy gums is acid reflux. Usually acid reflux- or GERD- will cause problems with the teeth- holes, cavities, breaking fillings, but I've also seen reflux cause red and swollen gums.

If this is you, you need to make sure that you see your doctor and try to control it. This acid will not only eat away your esophagus lining and cause ulcers, but it can cause ulcers in the mouth and also cavities.

The last culprit that I'll talk about is pop. We're in Ohio, we call it pop. Other parts of the country call it, soda, Coke, cola, soda pop.

Whatever, I don't care what you call it- I call it "instant holes in the teeth." I've seen teenagers drinking two liters of Mountain Dew- literally- in my office and wonder why they need 14 cavities filled. It's because you're drinking sugary acid. Most sodas' PH range from 3-4.

I'll never forget one family came in. They had just got back from the store and the dad came in with 4 cases of Pepsi and dropped them on the floor while I was checking his son for cavities.

I asked if that was their favorite pop and he said the whole family drank it and this should last them for the rest of the week. I just shook my head and as he said that, I noticed his two front teeth were black and rotted and that he was definitely missing a bunch of teeth.

I wanted to take a picture of him with his pop and make him my poster child for drinking that crap, but I didn't. And you know why? Because I felt bad for the guy when I gave him the bill for 22 fillings to fix his teenage son's teeth that were rotting to the core which was over $2500.

"Well, I like diet pop, isn't this better?"

Ok, you're not getting the sugar to provide food for the bacteria to eat and release acid that causes a cavity, you're just drinking pure acid that by itself will break down the enamel and cause cavities.

So no, it doesn't matter if it's naturally sweet acid or fake sweet acid, it's still horrible for your teeth. I haven't seen as many people with swollen and red gums from pop drinkers as I have tooth problems. So do me a favor, don't drink anything that has carbonation on a daily basis.

Sports drinks, carbonated waters, and sparkling drinks, none of it!

Your mouth will thank you!

CHAPTER 4

I WAKE UP WITH HEADACHES AND MY JAWS ARE SORE. WHAT IS WRONG WITH ME?

I see people all of the time that come in with different types of TMJ related symptoms. Sometimes their actual TMJ joint hurts, it's tense or sore.

Sometimes their teeth are sore when they wake up in the morning, like they've been clenching and biting on them during the night. Other times they come in with just plain headaches and want to know if there's anything that I can do to help them.

And the answer is yes, I can help in almost all of these instances.

According to the Migraine Research Foundation, over 40 million Americans suffer from migraine headaches. What most people don't know is that most headaches are not migraine headaches, but tension headaches. So what's the difference?

Migraine headaches are actually a neurologic storm that affects multiple nerves in the head. Most migraine headaches are associated with not only pain in the head and maybe neck, but also other symptoms like nausea, vomiting, dizziness, seeing stars in your vision, and light sensitivity.

So when there are multiple symptoms, that's a full blown migraine headache. I myself know when I'm going to have a migraine when I start seeing a flashing light in the corner of my eye.

Usually when this happens, I immediately take ibuprofen and drink some Gatorade which seems to help balance my electrolytes and help the migraine symptoms. Many times it goes away.

But I have had a migraine that has totally consumed my vision where I couldn't see and then my head started throbbing where I had to go to sleep until it wore off.

This has only occurred twice in my life but I know how debilitating that could be. I can't even imagine what it's like to have this occur on a frequent basis.

Prescriptive and non-prescription drugs and lifestyle changes can help to reduce the likelihood and frequency of migraines. But there's still no cure and not every therapy works on every person.

If this doesn't sound like your symptoms, then it's a tension headache. This is caused by some type of stress, from work, kids, or spouse issues.

I've seen multiple sales people who drive all day and deal with traffic issues that come in the office and say their neck, jaw, and head hurt all the time. Stupid traffic!

Anyways, usually tension headaches cause throbbing, tight pain that usually surrounds the temple areas on one or both sides of the head. It can make a radiating pain to the ear.

It can cause pain in the TMJ area and also cause the teeth to be sore. Sometimes a person can wake up in the morning and have tightness or soreness in their temple area or joint.

All of this can be caused by either clenching or grinding your teeth at night. This can have multiple effects on the head and neck areas.

One effect is that there's inflammation that can build up in the jaw joint itself. This can cause soreness and if the cartilage in the joint becomes damaged, a gravel, grinding, popping sound can occur when you open your mouth.

When the muscles of the head- mostly the temporalis muscle on the side of the temples- are being used all night- clenching or grinding away at the teeth- this is basically "working out" the muscle off and on all night.

Just like going to the gym and having a hard workout or doing something you haven't done in a while, this can build up lactic acid which accumulates in the muscles on the temple areas and can cause tightness or soreness.

It's like you've been working out all night! This inflammation and build-up of lactic acid can pinch off nerves and also signal chemicals that can cause a headache.

Another problem I see all the time that can trigger tension headaches is sleeping with a new pillow. This is usually the first thing I ask a patient who has never complained about grinding or headaches before and all of a sudden they come in to see me about having some monster headaches or their jaw is out of alignment.

If we sleep for years with the same pillow, what happens to the pillow? It gets flat. Then our body is used to the amount of tilt that the pillow creates on our head and neck and our body is used to that position during sleep. But what happens when you buy a new pillow?

It's large and fluffy and usually double the size of our old pillow. This can be good but it can also be bad. The good part is that the new pillow can help to put our head and neck in a more stable, neutral position where the head is not tilted down but more level with the neck.

But if the new pillow is very thick and fluffy, it can be more harm than good. In this case, it can turn the head upward, causing an upward slant to the head and neck. This can put a lot of pressure both on the neck vertebrae and also the TMJ area, possibly throwing the TMJ out of socket.

If you continue to sleep in this way, you will start feeling pain either in the joint, throughout the muscles of the head, neck pain, or any combination. And it won't go away unless you get rid of the new pillow or somehow smoosh it down so that your head and neck are again in a neutral, level position.

Usually this will take a couple of weeks for your body to heal itself and then all of a sudden, the pain goes away. This is definitely an acute problem that will go away just as fast as it started occurring.

Going along with this same theme is the stomach sleeper. This is usually the second thing that I ask people that come into my office with sudden headache/TMJ pain symptoms.

It's the same philosophy that goes along with the new pillow problem. When someone sleeps consistently on their stomach, it can put the neck, head, and especially the TMJ in a very awkward position.

Many times this can actually dislocate the TMJ slightly and can cause soreness in the joint, or surrounding muscles. This can also cause tension headaches.

If stomach sleepers quit the stomach sleeping and go back to sleeping on their back or side, usually these symptoms will go away by itself.

Anytime the TMJ area is tight and swollen, I tell my patients to use anti-inflammatories and also heat. Heat will help to relax the muscles. It's just like a sprain or pulled muscles.

You ice for the first 24 hours to try to constrict the blood vessels so that inflammation doesn't occur. But after 24 hours, there's already inflammation and trapped lactic acid so heat is then the best way to try to relax the muscles and increase blood flow which will then help to get rid of the lactic acid.

Most people that I see that have chronic tension headaches are either grinders or clenchers. When I diagnose them I first ask them about their symptoms.

First I ask about headaches- when do they occur. Usually this is the first thing in the morning or maybe the last thing at night. I also ask them if they have any popping or clicking in their jaw when they open their mouth.

Sometimes they do, sometimes they don't. When they do, this can mean that this has been happening over a long period of time and has caused damage inside the joint- usually to the cartilage that covers the joint.

I then ask them if there's any soreness or tightness in their temple muscles. As I've stated before, if these muscles are hyperactive all night long, they will become swollen and sore due to the lactic acid that the body produces when the cells don't have enough oxygen. Usually if they're clenching, they have soreness or tightness in these areas.

The next thing I look for is wear on their teeth. If they are just clenching, they usually won't have a lot of wear on the tops of the teeth. But if they're grinding at night- their teeth will be worn flat.

Our teeth are supposed to be pointy and lock themselves into each other like a puzzle. This helps to stabilize the jaw and train the muscles to put the lower jaw back in this particular place every time we close our mouths.

But if the teeth are flat, there's no particular place for the mouth to go and this can make the jaws slide around even worse at night, causing even more activity and soreness.

And people that don't have any back teeth- this problem can be even worse because there's no teeth to lock the jaws in place so all night long, their jaw is moving around trying to get itself into a comfortable spot.

So what can be done for the clencher/grinders of the world?

A simple mouth guard made by your dentist can help to eliminate the headaches, wear on the teeth, and soreness/tightness that all stems from an overactive jaw.

There are still some camps that make a mouth guard that covers either all the upper or lower teeth.

I'm in a camp that makes a mouth guard that only covers the front couple of teeth.

I've been making the NTI mouth guard for my patients for 15 years now and have seen hundreds and hundreds of patients become symptom free just by wearing this small device.

There are numerous YouTube videos about the NTI- even my own website has one- www.akrondentalconcepts.com/videos. Many dentists that are in my camp feel that if we engage the back molars, it can cause the clenching or grinding to be worse.

But if we make a small mouth guard that just keeps the mouth open slightly, disengaging the strong muscles near the back molar teeth, this will cause the patient to relax those back muscles, eliminating all the lactic acid and inflammation that occurs with overuse of those muscles.

My patients still grind or clench, but it's not as bad or strong and their headache symptoms usually go away within a few days. And although they're still grinding, they're grinding on my plastic mouth guard and not grinding on their own teeth, causing more wear and future problems with breakage and cold sensitivity from the lack of protective enamel.

So ask your dentist how they can prevent your headaches!

CHAPTER 5

WHY SHOULD I USE A SOFT TOOTHBRUSH? I DON'T FEEL LIKE IT CLEANS MY TEETH LIKE A MEDIUM ONE DOES

This is a constant struggle for my generation of dentists. We are fighting many factors that people face every day. We need to prevent cavities by removing plaque that contains food particles as well as bacteria that can release acids that can cause cavities.

But we must also conserve enamel which is our body's natural defense against the bacteria and their acids. And our gums are one of the last defenses to protect us against temperature sensitivity issues and also tooth loss and they are very sensitive to environmental changes such as abrasion and plaque accumulation.

So what is a person to do that wants to have the healthiest mouth ever? Use a soft or medium toothbrush? The true answer is none of the above. The true answer is to use an electric/rotary soft toothbrush.

These types of toothbrushes can greatly reduce the amount of plaque at the gum lines without putting too much pressure against the gums causing recession. Many electric toothbrushes on the market have built in sensors that will stop working if you're brushing too hard.

Electric toothbrushes apply a force of 80-150 g/f where manual toothbrushes/human strength can apply 250 g/f. That's a 40% reduction in the amount of force the toothpaste is pushed against the enamel and gums. Cool, right?

Major toothpastes on the market contain abrasives like Hydrated Silica, Hydrated Alumina, Calcium Carbonate, and Dicalcium

Phosphate. This can help clean the plaque off your teeth but it can also help to remove any organic stains that can build-up on the enamel surface, helping to "buff" out the enamel.

In a 2004 study by JL Forest and SA Miller in the Journal of Dental Hygiene, they showed that rotating, oscillating toothbrushes showed a 7% reduction in plaque and a 17% reduction in gingivitis- inflammation of the gums.

The Cochrane Oral Health Group reviewed 56 studies from 1964-2011 with 5068 participants which showed a 21% reduction of plaque after 3 months of use and 11% reduction in gingivitis after 3 months. Electric toothbrushes obviously help!

In my practice, my hygiene department has seen a significant reduction in plaque and tartar buildup with patients that use an electric toothbrush.

Most of the time that I do exams on these people that switch from manual to electric toothbrushes tell me that their visit to us was quicker and not as much "picking and scraping" as previous visits. I tell them that it's like buffing your car by hand or with an electric buffer- of course it will be more shiny and smoother if you use a rotary machine. It's just logical.

Most people brush for less than 1 minute. In this time a lot can be missed when doing it manually. If you use an electric toothbrush, it can get those areas 10 times more compared to just going over it once. It just makes common sense.

But for those out there that have to have their teeth shiny and smooth and want to use a medium toothbrush, PLEASE, PLEASE, PLEASE be careful!

You are forcing that abrasive toothpaste molecules against the enamel and gums and have a very high chance of causing wear and even gum loss/recession that will occur over time.

About 60% or more of my patients all have some type of gum recession- most of which are caused by either brushing too hard or by using a medium toothbrush.

These patients often complain about tooth sensitivity to cold and sometimes even touching their teeth they will get a "zing." These people don't realize that they have significantly reduced the amount of enamel that was protecting their tooth structure.

Enamel is a pretty solid surface. The next layer into the tooth is called dentin. This layer looks like Swiss cheese and inside those holes there's little tubes that house water.

Hot and cold temperatures can cause the water inside those tubes to contract and expand- this can cause the "zing" that people feel that have gum recession when cold things touch those areas. It can be quite uncomfortable and can cause these people to stop drinking and eating cold foods to try to avoid that pain.

There are several products on the market that can help reduce this water contraction in the dentin tubes. Products like Sensodyne or other sensitivity toothpastes contain Potassium Nitrate or Strontium Chloride.

These molecules help to block or cover up the exposed dentin tubes so that temperature changes nor abrasive actions can cause that water in those tubes to move and it decreases that pain or tooth "zing."

The only problem is that these molecules don't last very long. Your saliva washes them away over the course of the day so continuous use of these products is mandatory if you have tooth sensitivity from gum recession and wear and you want to keep it at a minimum.

Another form of treatment for gum recession is to cover that area up with a composite/white/plastic/bonded filling. I cover up hundreds of areas a year that have been worn down to the brink of exposing the nerve.

I usually monitor people's recession areas- the hygiene department will record yearly what these levels are and if we see that they are getting worse, I will jump in and put a filling over these areas. This does two things.

The first thing is the filling covers and blocks the exposed dentin tubes, thus reducing the water contraction and expansion that can occur from temperature fluctuations.

The second thing it does is give the tooth more bulk so that it's not so thin in that area and can relieve the constant abrasive forces of food against the gum line. I tell my patients that they can wear this filling out and if it gets thin and falls out, guess what?

I'll put another one in. At least they won't be wearing out their own tooth structure causing more damage. A filling I can replace very easily.

I have seen other treatments out there, but I haven't read any long term studies on them. There are some types of gum regeneration/ recontouring procedures, but this gets out of my league of expertise.

A gum surgeon or periodontist would know if there's any other options out there for people that have recession and don't want to use sensitive toothpastes for the rest of their lives or have bonding on their teeth done.

One of the major reasons why we need to preserve our gums is to prevent periodontal disease. What is periodontal disease? This disease is a slow resorption/destruction of the bone sockets that hold the teeth in place.

Usually this bone is very thin by the gum line and when the gums start to recede from over-brushing or using that medium toothbrush. When the gums go, the bone will start to go too eventually leading to loose teeth that will need to be taken out.

According to a 2006 study by the CDC, over 35 million Americans are over the age of 65. 25% of them no longer have their own teeth. Another 23% have severe periodontal disease- many at risk of losing whatever teeth they do have.

So over time, over half of us as we age will be wearing dentures by the time we're 65. This is awful! I know that many people of the baby boomer generation didn't have access to dental care when they were younger, nor were exposed to many state-wide water fluoride programs thus causing their tooth loss. But I know in my Generation X, the statistics for tooth loss will be caused by brushing too hard causing gum recession and bone loss.

So the bottom line is: Be nice to your gums! You don't need to use an expensive electric toothbrush, just get a cheap one! There are many different models and products on the market.

It will save your enamel. It will help to save your gums. It will help to save your bone that holds your teeth in your jaw. And it will help to save your teeth!

Trust me, nothing I can make for you will make you look as good and allow you to eat what you want like your own teeth! You only get 2 sets of them. Don't abuse your adult teeth. Baby them and they will keep you from eating baby food when you're older!

But if you do have sensitivity or any of the other problems that I've talked about in this chapter, make sure you come see me and talk to me about your options.

 Or if you don't live in my area, talk with your dentist about ways to prevent enamel loss, tooth sensitivity, and tooth loss! You'll be glad you did!

CHAPTER 6

WHY DO I HAVE TO FLOSS? THE HYGIENIST IS ALWAYS BUGGING ME ABOUT THIS.

This is a subject near and dear to my heart. Flossing. It's only string, right? I usually can tell if a person flosses or not when they come in the office for the first time after I check out their mouths. How? They usually have nice pink gums and very little fillings in their mouth.

So why do we harp on you some much to get that floss in between your teeth? Floss can benefit your mouth in two ways.

1. It will get the food out that's stuck between the teeth.

2. It will toughen up the gum tissue making it more resistance to gingivitis/inflammation.

So how does floss do this?

Floss brushes against those hard-to-reach spots in between the teeth where the toothbrush can't get to. The food and plaque that accumulates there is then dislodged from these surfaces, thus cleaning these surfaces. This can decrease tremendously the amount of bacteria and their acidic by-products that they release in this area.

These bacterial by-products are responsible for the breakdown of your enamel and can cause cavities. These bacterial by-products can also cause inflammation, redness, and bleeding of the little gum triangles in between your teeth called papilla.

When these triangles become agitated, they can start to breakdown themselves and the bone can go with it which is called recession.

The bacteria in our mouths love to eat the food that we love to eat. If there's big chunks of chicken stuck in between your teeth, the bacteria in your mouth have a huge party and release a ton of acid that starts to attack everything in sight- including your enamel and gum tissue.

Once this process starts, the enamel and gum tissue can only fight for so long, and then bad things happen- cavities and gum recession/ gingivitis.

So why not floss right before bed or after you've had a big meal to make sure that the bacteria in your mouth don't have their own sadistic party in your mouth? It's a simple task that will take you less than a minute to complete.

I know, I know, I hear all the stories every day.

I don't have time.

I have kids.

I can't get my man hands in my mouth.

I floss right before I come see my dentist.

My dog ate it.

I've heard it all.

But I just laugh and take everyone's money to have my hygienists pick and scrape all the junk that's collected on and in between their teeth. And then they complain because their mouth is bleeding and the cleaning hurt and they hate coming into the dentist.

And I just laugh again and take their money and set them up for another appointment in 4-6 months so that my team can do it all again because they simply didn't pick up a piece of floss and use it.

Ok, I need to pay for my kid to go to college and this is a super easy way to do it!

Besides getting the food and plaque out from in between the teeth, floss does another amazing thing. It helps to build up keratin in the gum tissue.

Keratin is like a callous on your finger. It's tougher and less prone to damage like Kevlon vests.

Think of the bacterial by-products as acidic bullets that want to penetrate your soft, pink, non-suspecting gum tissue. If you floss your teeth every day, over time your gum tissue will develop a bullet-proof vest that will help to wave off any bacterial by-products that come their way.

This will reduce the inflammation, redness, puffiness, and bleeding that's associated with gingivitis and will eventually result in periodontitis which is gum and bone loss resulting in your teeth falling out and you needing dentures! I know, scary thought, but all of this is true!

So besides painting a picture of ugly, gross bacteria eating the beef nachos that are stuck in between your teeth and having a party, here's another way I want to convince you to start flossing every day.

I was watching the Today show and happened to see one of the most ignorant reports I have ever seen on TV- and that's not saying much since the media shows us what they want us to see, not necessarily the whole story.

Anyways, the report was from the Associated Press and how they don't recommend flossing anymore due to the lack of scientific evidence.

Really?

Are there hundreds of research studies on the market that have studied that you should take a shower and make sure you wash every inch of your body?

Are there research studies out there that tell you to wash your clothes after wearing them during the day? Are there research studies that tell you to be careful handling paper because it can cause instant paper cuts?

No.

It's just common sense. We have 5 surfaces to our teeth- 1 top, and 4 sides. If one side is butting up to a side of another tooth, how can a toothbrush get in there to clean it?

That's right, it can't!

The only way to get the food and plaque out of that area is to put some floss in there that will catch the debris and remove it from in between your teeth.

Period!

I looked in my office computer and researched how many fillings I had done between 2000-2016 that included the surfaces in between the teeth?

Out of 16,354 fillings placed between March 17, 2000 and August 2, 2016, 9023 of those fillings involved the surfaces in between the teeth!

That's 55%!

So my patients have a 50/50 chance of needing a filling in between their teeth! And a simple solution to help combat this- floss once a day!

That's it! It's not that difficult!

I usually advise my patients to floss right before bed if they only have one time of day that they will do it. That way, their mouth is clean and free from food and debris that they shoved in their mouths during the entire day. It doesn't matter if you floss before or after you brush.

I like to floss before I brush because it seems like I get a lot of stuff out of my teeth and then I can buff out the other surfaces better. But I couldn't find any studies on how effective it is to brush before or after flossing. I just want people to floss.

That's a lot of fillings to be done on surfaces of the teeth that clearly don't get touched with brushing alone!

So what kind of floss should you use? In the U.S. the floss market is worth over $200 million every year. The Glide brand holds ½ of these sales and is made by Proctor and Gamble- the ones that make Crest products.

This is the kind of floss I use personally and have in my office. It's made out of Gore-Tex fibers which are pretty tough and resistant to tearing.

This is the same material they use for water proof coats. If you have tight teeth, have braces, or a lot of dental work in your mouth, this can cause cheap floss to tear and get stuck in your teeth.

The Glide floss usually can handle these conditions and will just slide in and out without getting stuck or causing further damage.

So how do I get this stuff in my mouth and floss properly? In dental school they told us to hold the floss between our two middle fingers- wrapping the floss around them and then we can use our thumbs and pointer fingers freely to get in and around our mouths to floss our teeth.

I use this every day on myself and the 40 people that I see every day. You don't want to put the floss in between the teeth and then see-saw it back and forth- this can cause cuts to the gum tissue and can cause bleeding and pain.

You want to get the floss in between the teeth and then gently go up and down and wrap the floss around the teeth so that it causes a sweeping motion on the teeth surfaces- this will dislodge any food and plaque that has accumulated in these areas and won't cause damage.

If you have a lot of dental work or braces, you would then just pull the floss through. You don't necessarily have to snap the floss back through the teeth again.

You can just snap it in, sweep the tooth surfaces, and then pull it back out. And then you're done!

Not so hard, now was it?

You take more time making your morning coffee, brushing your hair, and putting on makeup than it takes to floss your teeth once a day!

If you have big man hands or have trouble with your dexterity, there are numerous floss helpers on the market that can help you get that floss in the places it needs to go.

There are floss threaders that help to thread the floss under bridges and in between braces and retainers. There are dental picks that can help massage the gums and get stuff out of the triangle areas.

There are floss handles that have floss already on them that can help you reach those spots that aren't easy to get to. There are tiny triangular brushes that can get in between teeth and other dental work that you may have in your mouth. The possibilities are endless.

So please, please, please floss at least once a day!

You will love your dentist and hygienist if you do because you won't be seeing them very often to fix problems in your mouth!

But if you still won't do it, please come visit me- I need to pay for my retirement and my kid's college education and you will help me with that!

CHAPTER 7

I HAVE A 2 YEAR OLD THAT STILL HAS A BINKY. WHAT'S WRONG WITH THAT?

As a mother, I know that I have to sleep and to do this means that my child and my husband must be happy and tired and sleeping. But I also know that sometimes they can't always get what they want before they go to sleep. This includes a binkie or pacifier.

As a mother, I understand that all you want in your house is peace and quiet so you can actually think for 5 minutes. But as a dentist with over 8 years of college and 17 years of practice under my belt, this subject irritates the crap out of me!

Allowing your child who already has teeth in their mouth to suck constantly on a pacifier is just as bad as giving your child milk, pop, or juice in their bottles and sending them to bed! It can cause a lot of damage.

And thumb sucking is worse because you can take the pacifier away but a thumb unfortunately is attached and goes with your child wherever they go.

So why am I so irritated with the whole binkie thing? As an infant, our precious little bundles of joy have a natural instinct to suckle.

They want to have milk from mommy. This suckling effect helps to soothe and comfort them when they come into this crazy, noisy world.

This isn't a problem.

A pacifier can certainly help with promoting this natural instinct and can help put your baby in a relaxed state. Which usually means that you as the mommy or daddy can have some relaxation too.

But when your child is 3 and is demanding something to eat and is walking around singing, and dancing, and sucking on a pacifier, this is when the problem starts! My own family members laughed and scoffed at me when I told them I didn't want my child to have a binkie.

I actually caved in when he was first born and he used a pacifier for a couple of weeks and then he didn't want it anymore and I didn't back down and return it to him.

And to this day, I still have family members having problems with their children's teeth being messed up and they're walking around with binkies in their mouths. Needless to say, I know a little bit more on the subject than some of them. But I digress....

In the January/February 2007 issue of General Dentistry from the Academy of General Dentistry,

"Prolonged pacifier use and thumb sucking can cause problems with the proper growth of the mouth, alignment of the teeth and changes in the shape of the roof of the mouth," says AGD spokesperson Luke Matranga, DDS, MAGD, ABGD.

During orthodontic movement of the teeth, a safe amount of force to put on the teeth without damaging the roots or surrounding bone is about 2 ounces or the weight of 2 pieces of bread- not very hard at all.

When your child is chewing their pacifier, they are exuding forces similar to the forces of a dog bite. In a 2009 study from the University of Leeds, they studied the bite strengths of 200 children and found that some of the children exuded bite strength similar to that of a dog- 235-328 pounds of pressure.

Pounds of pressure- not ounces of pressure. Have you ever put your finger in your child's mouth and quickly wished you hadn't as they chomped down on your finger as you cried out in pain? You know how strong those little jaws are.

And now you're putting a piece of rubber in their mouths that they will put over 200 pounds of pressure over and over and over again on these poor little baby teeth. Of course they're going to move and chip and break. And their poor little mouths.

The roof of their mouths become elongated and look like a "V." And usually they have an open bite. This means that they will close their teeth together in the back, but their palates are so stretched out and up that their front teeth don't meet and you could stick a block in between their teeth in the front and still have their back teeth touching.

This is not a situation that an orthodontist can easily fix when they're teenagers. The damage is already done.

I know that we as parents want to make our kids happy. I get that. But we make them take baths. We make them eat their vegetables.

We make them brush their teeth and hair. Why do we allow them to run around with pacifiers when it's clinically known to damage their mouths and teeth?

This is definitely a battle that is worth fighting. And the same thing goes with thumb sucking.

I know that it's also a soothing method but it causes the same amount of damage to their teeth and palates.

STOP THE MADNESS!

When your child doesn't have any teeth, a pacifier is a suitable thing to use to soothe your child. Up until the age of 2 when they have all of their baby teeth, any problems with alignment of their teeth or the developing palatal bone is usually corrected within a 6-month period after the binkie or thumb is discontinued.

But after the age of 2, the teeth and palate are more formed and are more difficult to correct with continued use of the pacifier.

So what's a parent to do to stop this habit? In the case of the binkie- it's simple. Throw it out!

Trust me, you're in control of the situation. Your child can't get in the car and drive to the store and get another one.

They don't have a choice in this matter. Take control of the situation and get rid of it. If you want to ease it from them, put a small hole in it.

Over the course of a few days, make the hole bigger. This will get rid of the pressure that the pacifier creates and it won't be appealing to the child anymore. I've have numerous patients try this and have it work for them over the years.

Pacifiers are a lot easier to control than thumb sucking. And the older the child is when you are attempting to change his/her behavior, the harder it is.

Some experts recommend vinegar, hot sauce, or cinnamon to put on their thumb nails to help deter their habit. They make a bitter nail polish for those kids that bite their nails that can help.

If the child is old enough to handle a reward system, other experts say to reward them with a toy or an experience if they go 7 days without sucking their thumbs.

Most experts in pediatrics say that thumb sucking habits can stop by the age of 5 on their own accord, but if your child is still doing this by kindergarten, they can not only suffer mouth issues, but can be teased by those mean other kids in their class.

Thumb suckers can also have chapped skin, calluses, and other infections involving their thumbs. I remember my own sister had a huge red sore on her finger for a long time because she couldn't keep her thumb out of her mouth.

Some pediatricians suggest a sock placed over their hand and tied with ribbon or a shoelace. This will prevent the thumb flexibility that the child is used to and they won't be able to put it in their mouth as easily.

There are also retainers that your orthodontist can make that can deter that thumb from going in your child's mouth- mostly taking up the palatal space that the thumb occupies.

If there's no room in their mouth for their thumb, the habit can go away quickly. You know your child. You know what works, but it's your responsibility to take control of the situation and stop this horrible habit that will have dire consequences to their speech and eating abilities in the future.

You can do it!

Take no prisoners and don't negotiate with the terrorists, I mean children!

CHAPTER 8

I GOT ALL MY TEETH OUT AND THESE DENTURES ARE ALL OVER THE PLACE. WHAT ARE MY OPTIONS TO FIX THIS?

There are a few ways to help fix a "floppy denture" and these depend on several factors including:

1. How old you were when you got your teeth out.
2. How bad was your bone loss before you got your teeth out?
3. If we're talking about a lower or upper denture
4. Your health conditions

Let's tackle each one independently. The first and second factors have to do with the age you were when you got your teeth out.

Typically, the newer the denture, the more jaw bone height and width is available to use to balance the denture on. After the teeth are taken out, there's holes where the teeth were living in the jaw bones.

These holes are called sockets. After the teeth are taken out, the sockets usually partially collapse on the thin sides and the bone fills in the remaining hole. This means you automatically lose at least 30% of the bone as soon as the teeth are out of the jaws.

After the bone heals- which typically takes six months to a year to complete, it is already shorter and thinner than it was when there were teeth present.

Then add the factor of aging, especially females who tend to have Vitamin D and Calcium issues after the age of 35, and this can also cause resorption of the bone, making it thinner and shorter.

Then add other factors like smoking, Diabetes, and other health conditions and medications that can affect the bone height and width and you've got yourself a floppy denture.

Knowing how these factors can affect a piece of plastic with teeth on it, I always encourage my patients to try to keep as many teeth in their mouths as possible.

It's a lot easier to make partial dentures that can be secured in their mouths by existing teeth and bone height and width than by using suction and stability only.

Those existing teeth can help to stabilize the partial denture and can allow the patient to eat and talk more naturally because they feel the security of the appliance in their mouth. Full dentures need more help.

Another factor to consider is if we're talking about an upper denture or a lower denture. Usually an upper denture incorporates the palate which has a lot of thin tissue on it that when moist can create a suction power that helps to keep the denture in place.

Top this off with some denture adhesive cream and this upper denture can be pretty stable. However there are some drawbacks to an upper denture. One of which is the covered palate.

There are some taste buds in this soft palatal tissue and most people that wear a full upper denture complain that they don't taste their foods the same as when they had teeth. And this is one of the reasons why.

Another drawback to a full upper denture is that some people are naturally "gaggy" people. They can't take pills easily. They often have either small mouths, big tongues, small airways, or a combination.

I have one patient that I am the only one that can clean her teeth or do any work on her. I look at her and she begins to gag. Over the years, I've developed strategies and methods that I use just on her to make her feel at ease and to not awaken her gag demon.

I don't even want to think about what she would be like if we had to make her a full upper denture. It probably wouldn't happen.

For those "gaggy" patients, you can shorten the denture, but sometimes when you do this, you break the natural seal that the denture makes with the hard and soft palate.

At the border of the hard and soft palate, a lot of suction can be created. If you trim this area and only secure the denture to the hard palate, you lose the suction in this area.

But sometimes you have to compromise on this- either you wear it with some paste to help create the suction and keep it in your mouth or you constantly gag and throw up every time you try to wear it. Obviously the latter situation wouldn't go very far.

If we're talking about a lower denture, this is a whole different story. For one thing, you have a tongue that is constantly moving and potentially lifting up the lower denture.

You can only build the U-shaped denture that sits on the ridge- or lack of. If there's no height or width to this ridge, then the denture is going to rest on the surrounding tissue and muscles which attach to the sides of the ridge.

So every time you talk or chew you'll be using these muscles which will affect the position of the denture and can make it move and flop around in your mouth.

Denture adhesives can again help to stabilize the lower denture. But they are messy and will harbor bacteria if not fully cleaned daily.

The lower denture usually is the big problem for patients. The upper one they usually can get used to very quickly. But there's another solution to a floppy lower denture and we'll get into that in a bit.

But for now, we want to look at different factors that could cause a floppy denture.

The last factor that can cause problems is your health condition. If you have certain health conditions such as Parkinson's, Lupus, Diabetes, Sjogren's, or Reflux/GERD, these can all cause dry mouth conditions which can decrease the amount of saliva in your mouth and can decrease the suction power the saliva plays with the soft tissues in your mouth and the plastic denture.

Over 500 medications - some prescription and some over-the-counter can also cause dry mouth. We get into this a lot more in the chapter about dry mouth problems.

So the next question is what do you do if you have a health condition, take a dry-mouth-producing medication, had your teeth out when you were young, don't have a lot of bone to hold the denture in place, and have floppy dentures?

Well, there's two things that can be done to help stabilize those dentures. One way is to reline the denture.

There are two different types of reline materials. There's a soft reline material and there's a hard reline material. I only use the hard reline material and here's why.

The soft reline material is only soft for about two weeks and then it will start drying out and will become harder. But it's still soft enough that parts of it could break off and can cause more food to get stuck in the denture or will hurt the seal that's created because part of it is missing.

It can also harbor more bacteria in the pores of the material and can cause a bad odor and also secondary infections if a sore is made for a poor fitting denture.

For a hard reline, an impression must be taken with the loose denture and then sent to the lab for the day. The dental lab will then flow hard acrylic material- the same material that the denture is made from- and will fill in any gaps that may occur between the denture and the soft tissue of the mouth.

If you lose a lot of weight, have dry mouth because of a health condition or from a medication, this can affect the plumpness of the soft tissues in the mouth and this can cause a loose denture.

In these instances, a hard reline will help with stability and retention of the denture.

If a weight issue nor a dry mouth issue is causing your denture to flop around in your mouth, it may be from the lack of bone height and width which we mentioned earlier.

In this case, the only hope to stabilize your denture is with dental implants. What are dental implants and how do they stabilize your denture? Good questions!

Dental implants are titanium screws that go into your jaw and act like your teeth. So they have two parts. One is in the bone, the other sticks out of the bone and a snap is placed on it so that the snap on the denture can hold it in place.

It's very simple. The only thing that determines whether this will work or not is do you have enough bone to hold the implant and are you healthy enough to have the implants heal?

Bone takes 4-6 months to heal around implants depending on how much bone there is and the firmness of the bone. The lower jaw is very dense and usually takes around 4 months to heal while the upper jaw bone is more porous and can take up to 6 months to heal around an implant.

If you smoke, use tobacco products, have Diabetes, have heart issues that require blood thinners, these are all conditions that may take the bone longer to heal. Taking bisphosphonates can also affect how the bone heals and implants may even be contraindicated for people with these conditions.

Dental implants have a 98% success rate as long as the bone heals around them and stays healthy. I've had a couple of patients who had implants successfully for 20 years and have recently lost them due to poor health and poor hygiene.

If that bacteria from your mouth integrates in the bone near the junction of the implant/bone interface, this can damage that bone and the implants can fail.

So proper trips to your dentist is essential to keeping those implants clean and free of tartar and plaque buildup. Usually the people that have dentures are the same ones that had a lot of dental work done during their lives.

They either have poor hygiene, poor enamel, poor health, or a combination of one or more conditions. If one is to have implants placed to keep their denture snapped in, one must have great hygiene and keep themselves as healthy as possible.

There are many types of implants on the market and there's many general dentists and specialists that are trained to do these types of procedures. In my office I have been trained to do the mini implants as well as the traditional larger implants.

Mini implants are one piece very thin diameter implants. These implants work best to hold in lower dentures on patients with poor height and width of their lower jaws, and for patients that are congenitally missing a tooth from birth after braces are removed.

We also place traditional implants which are implants that have 2 parts- one in the bone, and one that sticks out of the gum to either snap a denture in place, or glue a crown or bridge on.

I tend to use the biggest implant system I can get into that bone. If they don't have a lot of bone, then the mini system is great. If they have some bone, a traditional implant system is the course of action!

When you're ready to know what option is right for you, ask your dentist. If they don't do the relines or the implant surgeries, have them refer you to either a gum surgeon/periodontist or an oral surgeon.

They can then see what type of system is best for you. Usually they will take a CBCT/3 D scan of your jaw and see in 3 dimensions where the bone is and how much is there so they can recommend the best course of treatment to snap in your denture. Normally a lower denture will require 2-4 implants while the upper denture would require 4-6 implants.

The reason a lower can have fewer is because the lower jaw bone is more dense and can handle the eating/chewing forces easier than the porous upper jaw bone.

So first, see if you need a reline. It's easy and a lot cheaper to see if that denture can have a snugger fit.

If you don't have a lot of bone to hold the denture, mini or traditional implants are the best treatment to help snap those dentures in your mouth and keep them from flopping around as long as your health and your habits are in decent shape.

You can check out videos about different procedure discussed in this book by going to my website www.akrondentalconcepts.com.

CHAPTER 9

WHAT ARE THE CONSEQUENCES OF HAVING A DRY MOUTH?

Saliva is an essential liquid in our body. It helps lubricate our tongue and soft tissue. It helps to neutralize the acids from foods and from the bacteria in our mouths.

It helps us swallow our food. It helps to supply Calcium and Phosphorous that helps to build enamel. It also helps to coat our tongues for taste perception.

So why don't I have a lot of saliva? My mouth is always dry?

To understand this, we need to know what can cause dry mouth, often referred to as Xerostomia. These days most symptoms of dry mouth are caused by 3 things including medications, medical conditions, and lifestyle habits.

Over 500 medications have "dry mouth" as a side effect. These can include antidepressants, decongestants, antihistamines, muscle relaxants, appetite suppressants, sedatives, non-steroidal anti-inflammatories, and diuretics.

I know, it's a lot.

That extends the market from Benadryl to Advil (over the counter drugs) and from Prozac to thiazides for high blood pressure (prescription drugs.)

Most drugs solve one problem and cause even more symptoms.

There's also medical conditions that can also cause a dry mouth including Diabetes (21 million in the USA), Scleroderma (300,000 in the USA), Parkinson's disease (60,000 in the USA), Sjogren's syndrome (4 million in the USA), Lupus (1.5 million in the USA), GERD (7 million in the USA), cancer patients (20 million in the USA) and Alzheimer's (5.4 million in the USA) which account for over 59 million people.

That's a third of the country!

Their conditions can affect the salivary flow in their mouths but then if they take medications to help the symptoms of these diseases, it's even worse.

The third cause of a dry mouth are lifestyle habits which include mouth breathing, smoking, chewing tobacco, caffeine, and alcohol use.

Nicotine and caffeine are both diuretics which basically cause the kidneys to increase the amount of salt and water that come out through the urine. Because of this disturbance in the natural flow of water through your body, your salivary glands can also be affected and will produce less saliva.

So the question is- so what? Who cares? Why is saliva so important in your life?

There are 6 main functions of saliva.

The first one is to help you speak, eat, and digest food. Saliva has natural enzymes called Amylase and Ptyalin which starts the breakdown of starches into simpler sugars such as Maltose and Dextrin that can be broken down in the small intestine.

If your food's digestion isn't broken down initially by saliva, your small intestine has to work much harder to break down your food.

Another function of saliva has to do with maintaining the PH of your mouth. The bacteria in your mouth release acid along with acidic foods that you eat.

Saliva not only helps to wash away this acidic foods and bi-products but it also helps to prevent gingivitis, periodontitis, and cavities.

Saliva also contains lysozymes, Peroxidase, and Lactoferrin which help to kill bacteria that enters your mouth.

Saliva helps to supply Calcium and Phosphorous to help build enamel which is one of the hardest substances in the body. Without newly repaired enamel, your teeth would soon develop holes and would eventually need pulled out.

Sometimes this still happens because the enamel is damaged from trauma, eating hard crunchy foods causing fractures, or eating sugary foods which cause the bacteria in your mouth to release more acid.

When this happens, your body can't repair itself fast enough and a hole/cavity occurs. This can then lead to tooth aches and eventually loss of the tooth or more extensive dental treatments like root canals and crowns.

Saliva helps to lubricate the mouth, tongue, and throat to allow food to move down the esophagus. This lubrication is also needed to talk and move your tongue and cheeks around.

Without it, things would be quite ugly in there! People with upper dentures also need saliva in their mouths to cause suction to help hold their upper dentures in place.

Gravity can be an awful thing for denture wearers! That's why we have Fixodent and other adhesives on the market- with so many adults having dry mouths, there's a strong need for denture adhesives to help keep their dentures in their mouths and not in their laps!

Without saliva, our tongues can't taste our foods. Saliva helps to coat the tongue and start the breakdown of foods which the taste buds signal as taste sensations.

Do you remember when you had a cold and you were on decongestants? How was your taste ability? Pretty lousy, huh?

That's because you had a dry mouth and there was no saliva to start the digestion of your food and your nose couldn't send any of its signals to the brain to interpret the smell and taste of that particular piece of food.

If someone has radiation or chemotherapy, its main purpose is to kill all rapidly dividing cells. This includes cancer cells but the goal is to not kill enough of the good cells that the body can fight the bad stuff and allow the cancer patient to live.

 The problem with these treatments is that is can also kill other cells like salivary glands and hair follicles- that's why chemotherapy patients lose their hair- it destroys the follicles and their mouths are very dry.

Finally, our saliva contains the IgA antibodies which are the first line of defense in our immune systems. IgA antibodies are produced in the mucous membranes.

These antibodies can also survive in our intestinal tract and can help maintain our gut health. If your salivary glands are damaged from either cancer treatments, medical conditions mentioned above, or medications they won't produce the IGA antibodies your body needs to fight infection!

Also if you have an ulcer or have a tooth taken out, saliva helps to increase wound contraction and clotting.

You didn't know saliva was so important, did you?

So the next question is- how do you keep your mouth moist when you're on medications or have a condition that causes dry mouth symptoms?

There's a couple of things you can do to keep your mouth moist. One is to drink lots of water. I know, everyone says that, but most people drink everything but plain, clear, non-tasting water.

Nowadays, people drink lots of lattes and mocha-china-type drinks all of which are high in Caffeine which is a diuretic. Sports drinks which are high in Sodium and other minerals are now a common "during the day" drink for people even if they didn't work out. These types of drinks aren't meant to be a part of your every day diet.

Also everyone drinks some type of pop/soda every day because they want the sweets. But again, a lot of these drinks contain Caffeine which will cause dry mouth symptoms.

They also can contain sugar and their PH are very acidic- so there's a triple whammy when it comes to pop/soda.

Alcohol and smoking can also act as diuretics causing dry mouth symptoms.

The bottom line is that drinking "Plain-Jane" water is a great prevention/solution to dry mouth symptoms no matter what they are caused from. I'm actually drinking a tall glass of water as I'm writing this chapter- it made me thirsty for some reason!

For people that have consistent dry mouth, there are product lines such as Biotene products, Spry chewing gum, Xylimelts, and Therabreath to name a few. Most of these products are over-the-counter but you still may need to ask your pharmacist for help finding these products. Their purpose is to stimulate saliva, help with lubrication of the mouth, and to help neutralize the acidic environment in the mouth.

Another defense against these secondary conditions is regular check-ups with your dentist. Talk to him/her about your concerns and make sure you catch things when they are small!

You'll thank your tooth and your wallet when things are fixed early!

CHAPTER 10

I HAVE A CHIPPED FRONT TOOTH AND THE FILLING KEEPS COMING OUT. WHAT'S THE MATTER?

This is a tough problem to fix. Once a tooth breaks, there's only 4 acceptable materials we as dentists can use to fix your teeth. One is porcelain which is basically glass. The second one is bonding composite which is basically plastic. The third is gold and the last one is silver amalgam.

So to fix a front tooth, there's only two appropriate materials to use- porcelain and composite bonding.

Most people choose the composite bonding because there's not a lot of tooth structure missing- it's usually just a chip in the tooth, and composite bonding material isn't as expensive as porcelain restorations such as crowns or veneers.

So why does the composite keep breaking off? We've got to look a little at the forces that play a role in your mouth. If you chip any tooth's tip or edge, the cheapest way to fix your tooth is to bond or glue plastic composite on the tooth surface.

As we've discussed throughout this book, the compressive strength of plastic composite bonding material is 250 mPa while the strength of tooth enamel is 384 mPa. This means that the plastic composite bonding material will flex more than the tooth structure.

If that plastic composite bonding material is only "stuck" on the edge of the tooth structure because that's where the tooth broke, there's no other support for that filling except that small junction of glue that is holding that flexible material onto the tooth structure.

If you're eating something hard like an apple or biting into a thick sandwich, this force will cause the composite bonding to flex and the force may be too much for the composite bonding to handle and it will crack off.

Think of a nail that's just barely into some wood. It's just stuck on the surface. If you tug even gently on the nail, it will come out of the wood. Composite bonding is just like this. It's just "stuck" on the surface.

I always tell my patients that these are the hardest fillings to keep in their mouths. Whether it's a top or bottom front tooth, if there's no tooth structure to help hold that filling in place- that it's just "stuck" to the broken edge of the tooth, the filling usually won't hold up over a long period of time and it will need to be redone.

When I do these type of teeth, I usually bulk up the filling material so it's a little thicker to help it stay in place. But sometimes people's bites are difficult to do this to and the material's thin in that area. I usually tell them in this instance that it will need to be redone and it could be often or we need to look into porcelain restorations.

So can we use porcelain instead? This depends on how big of a filling you need. To use porcelain, you have to have a thickness of at least .3mm.

And this is for thin porcelain like a veneer for example. But you also have to prep a veneer entirely on the outside of the tooth, in between the teeth slightly, and wrap around to the back side of the tooth's edge.

Do you need this much prepping of the tooth structure to fix your problem?

I hate shaving down good tooth structure just to make room for a certain filling material, but sometimes this is the only option to fix the tooth correctly.

If there's more than ⅓ of the tooth structure gone, then doing a porcelain veneer can help solve your problem. If there's less that

⅓ tooth structure gone, usually a composite bonded filling is all you need to fix the hole.

If there's more than that- often a crown will be needed to rebuild the tooth properly.

But it really depends on your eating habits- are you biting into foods like apples and corn on the cob? If you are, then a veneer or crown made from porcelain will have the strength similar to enamel- around 360 mPa- to be able to handle those types of forces.

But, and I say again- but, you still can break porcelain because it's only glass. If you flex that tooth enough, you can also break the porcelain.

When I first started doing dentistry, I remember doing a brand new porcelain crown on a friend's two front teeth. I specifically told him not to eat any hard foods for fear that it could break.

That weekend I was at a picnic with a bunch of people and saw my friend eating an apple. Low and behold he saw me the next week- he had accidentally fractured one of the crowns in half by biting into that apple.

I was so mad but this confirmed my belief in not putting too much pressure on any dental material that is used.

Remember that there's no substitute for your own enamel! So be careful. The softer your diet is, the less visits to the dentist for repair work you will incur.

 Now this doesn't mean that you have to eat baby food or get a blender and puree everything. This just means that your teeth are precious and you have to take care of them.

Let someone else eat those hard kettle chips, jaw breakers, ice cubes! Let them spend hundreds or thousands of dollars fixing up their teeth. Be smarter and eat softer stuff!

CHAPTER 11

DURING MY CHECK-UP, THE HYGIENIST AND DENTIST TALK ABOUT DIFFERENT THINGS. WHAT DO THEY MEAN?

These are certainly very important questions that need to be addressed every single time you see your dentist- or anyone for that matter!

Whether it's getting your car fixed, to doing a routine check up on your furnace to removing a crack that is forming in your tooth, a clear definition of what is wrong and why and when it should be fixed should be addressed.

So let's dive into the dental world again and talk about some things that could be mentioned at a routine dental cleaning/check-up that should make you aware that action may need to be taken sooner rather than later.

One such thing that the dentist or hygienist may bring up is the fact that you have bleeding gums. Ok, we know that most people don't floss their teeth on a routine basis.

Ok, I get it.

You're busy, you barely have enough time to actually brush them.

But what most people don't realize is the toothbrush only gets on the surfaces that we can actually see and doesn't do anything for the surfaces that are in between the teeth where they touch each other.

And if you have crooked teeth, the surfaces that don't get cleaned are even bigger and pose a high threat of cavities and disease in those areas.

Yes, I said disease.

Periodontal disease and dental decay are serious diseases that can have lifelong consequences that can affect the rest of your body and how it functions.

So we discussed earlier in Chapter 6 about flossing and its importance. If you're not flossing, usually there's a lot of buildup around your teeth and when the hygienists get in there to clean you up with their sharp metal instruments, your mouth bleeds and looks like a police homicide crime scene.

If the bacteria and their acidic by-products keep damaging the flimsy gum tissue- it will decide to go bye-bye and you will get recession and also when the gums recede, the bone goes with it causing periodontal disease bone loss.

When the bone recedes, you don't have as much bone surrounding your teeth and they get loose and will eventually fall out or need to be taken out.

It's a vicious cycle. But it's important to have great home care-brushing at least twice a day and flossing at least right before bed. So when you go in for your cleaning, listen to the report that the hygienist gives to the dentist so that you'll know if you need to bump up your level of care at home and avoid the progression of the periodontal disease that you have starting.

It's just like anything else- your body takes maintenance. In your younger days, you don't need to watch what you eat. You're always eating anything you want and never gain weight.

Then you go to college, drink too much and eat the wrong stuff- all of a sudden, you gain the "Freshman 15." Then you either realize that you need to change your ways, or you keep getting fatter and fatter and more and more out of shape. There's really only two things to do- correct the problem, or live with it.

The health of your mouth- your teeth and your gums are the same thing. In your 20's, you may have never had a cavity in your life.

Great! That's awesome!

But after practicing over 17 years, I can tell you, that only a small percentage of my patients are cavity-free by the time they are 30! And we live in an age where there's tons of medicines and supplements on the market, but you still have to physically brush and floss your teeth to get rid of the food and plaque that builds up on them over the course of the day.

And women especially are susceptible to decay and gum problems after having kids. Those precious little ones rob your body of key nutrients for months during pregnancy, and if you breastfeed, for months after. I've seen women have at least one cavity after each child they conceive. A scary thought!

It takes real effort to stay in shape, to cook healthy meals, to brush and floss your teeth every day. I've got my son- who's 5 right now, brushing and flossing!

We do it together in the morning before school and at night before we go to bed. I figured that good habits start at a young age and hopefully he can keep his smile healthy until he dies!

Another area that goes along with bleeding gums is your overall periodontal health. How healthy are your gums? This can be evaluated by looking at the condition of your gums. Are they pink and plump? Are they red and irritated? Do they fill in the areas between your teeth? Are they flappy?

Your periodontal health can also be tested by doing a probing depth. The gum tissue that's beside your teeth should have a depth measurement of between 1-3 mm.

Usually the front teeth will have tighter gums of 1-2 mm and the back teeth will have thicker gums of 2-3mm. Once you start getting 4mm and beyond, this means that the bone and gums aren't attached at the edges of the teeth anymore and they are starting to go down/up the roots.

When this happens, you will get recession and bone loss which can cause the teeth to become loose and eventually fall out or need to be taken out.

So listen to these readings- usually the hygienist will only tell the dentist the areas that have higher readings which may or may not be addressed.

Usually if the readings are a little higher, but there's no bleeding in these areas when they are probed, that usually indicates that there's no active disease in this area- all the damage has been in the past and now it's being maintained.

But if there's a lot of bleeding- this means the gums are being beat up and that things may get worse. Either special mouth rinses, increased home care, or supplementation may need to be stressed to inactivate this damaging process.

The next thing to listen for is wear on your teeth. If you are grinding your teeth, which you may or may not be aware of, you are mechanically getting rid of your enamel.

And once the enamel is gone, it is gone forever. This can lead to cold sensitivity, cavities, cracks in the teeth, and shorter teeth which can be hard for your dentist to fix.

A simple solution for this problem is to wear a mouth guard. This mouth guard can be custom made by your dentist or one that you can buy online or at the store.

Most store bought mouth guards are made from either plastic or a rubber material and can help to prevent you from grinding your teeth together at night. But sometimes these products make the problem worse because they are not fitted to your mouth and move around too much when you sleep.

This is where custom mouth guards can help. Your dentist can either take an impression of your mouth and send it away to a lab for them to make or your dentist can make it in their office. There's a lot of different designs for mouth guards out there.

Some cover all the teeth- either the upper arch or the lower arch. Some only cover the front teeth. I use the NTI bite splint that only covers the front few teeth.

This stops your mouth from closing all the way and you can still grind, but you'll be grinding on your mouth guard and not your own teeth!

The NTI not only helps grinding issues, but it also is FDA approved to help decrease the likelihood of headaches. Some people grind or clench so much at night that they build up lactic acid in their TMJ areas causing jaw soreness and tension headaches.

Make sure that your hygienist is checking on your TMJ area too- he/she will ask you some questions about grinding, headaches, or muscle soreness that may occur at night. This TMJ evaluation can go along with wear on your teeth.

Another area your hygienist will evaluate is old fillings that have either staining or defective edges. Composite plastic fillings can very easily start to leak.

By eating crunchy foods or from grinding your teeth at night, you can stress the bonded edges of your filling and this bond will eventually break.

Sometimes this break is very minimal but usually we will start seeing brown staining- usually from food and dark drinks that will accumulate in these areas. If the edges still feel sealed, the dentist may "watch" these areas and see if they get worse. If they do, the filling would have to be replaced. If not, nothing would be done.

If there's old silver amalgam fillings, over time the thin, straight edges can become worn. Usually these edges will then look thick and rolled.

Usually when I see this, I redo the filling. These rolled edges usually are openings for bacteria and their by-products to get under the filling and can rot the tooth from the inside out. I've seen this before.

I usually don't mess around when I see an old filling that has defective edges- I'd rather get to it now, than let it fester and get worse.

Another item that the hygienist is checking for is dark stains in the grooves of the teeth. We all have hundreds of tiny grooves in our teeth that help to collect our food and cause friction with our other teeth to chew and break down our food so we can digest it. But what happens when stain starts to accumulate in these areas?

Our enamel isn't the same thickness throughout our teeth. Our molars, for example, have thicker enamel at the cusp tips and in between our teeth. But at the gum line, the enamel becomes thin and also in the grooves.

If there's organic stain that collects in these fine lines, they can act like Velcro and attract more bacteria and food and can cause this enamel to become stressed and "viola"- a cavity will form.

I have some patients that drink a lot of coffee and tea and have stain in their grooves and have never had a problem nor a cavity.

And then I have other patients that start accumulating stain and then their enamel gives up and a cavity starts. This is why we take X-rays- we can usually see if the enamel in these areas are still strong or if it's starting to become a problem requiring a filling.

A general area that your hygienist will look at is your medical history. If your medications have changed can greatly impact the health of your mouth.

As we talked about in Chapter 9 about a dry mouth and the havoc that can play not only on your mouth but your overall digestive system. Medications and certain health conditions can also affect your dental treatment.

Let's say for instance that you are on a blood thinner. If you need a tooth taken out, this is a big red flag in my office and I will send you out to an oral surgeon.

When we take teeth out on people taking blood thinners, it can become difficult to control the bleeding in the extraction site and of course we don't want people bleeding to death from a little tooth extraction- right?

Other issues like allergies, sensitivities to metal, and heart conditions can affect dental treatment. As long as you fill out your medical history correctly and your list of medications, your hygienist and dentist can treat you appropriately.

Getting back to teeth issues- another topic of discussion should be cracks or hairline fractures in your teeth. As we eat hard foods or get a soccer ball to our face, we can develop tiny fractures in our teeth.

 Some of them are small and only on the surface of the enamel, but then there's others that are deeper and go past our enamel into deeper parts of our teeth and can cause pain, temperature sensitivity, and biting pressure. Both of these need to be addressed.

Usually when I shine light through someone's teeth, I can see tiny cracks in them- sometimes they are clear and tooth colored, sometimes they start collecting stain and become dark. Usually the light, clear ones, I watch.

These tend to be surface cracks and usually don't cause any problems with normal eating and trauma-free living. But the ones that start to collect stain and have irregular edges I always fix. Sometimes these fractures are beside a silver metal filling.

Depending on how big and how many of these cracks show up, I will either extend the filling into the cracked area or I recommend we do a crown on it to protect what's left of the shell of the tooth.

If these dark stained cracks are left alone, usually they get worse and either cause the tooth to break off, or worse, travel straight into the nerve, causing pain and infection that needs either extraction or a root canal.

As we've discussed throughout this book, it's a lot easier to get a filling done or a crown when it doesn't hurt than to have pain on the weekend or holiday, not be able to get in right away, and have to double the cost of doing a root canal and a crown or even worse, lose the tooth.

I always vote for the simple solution- and I do these all of the time. When I see a fracture line, if it's stained- I tell the patient that we should get rid of this crack and extend the filling or even do a crown so it doesn't get worse.

Most of the time this solves the problem and is a fast and cheap way of getting ahead of it.

Another observation the hygienist and dentist will make is if there's dark or white spots anywhere on the teeth- near the gum line, or on the biting surface.

These areas are decalcification areas. Basically what this means is that the Calcium and other minerals that help to build enamel are not plentiful in that area.

Those areas can easily be weakened by eating crunchy or acidic foods (pop or citrus) and can become what I call "potholes" in the enamel. If the enamel is still solid but there's marks on it- then we have a fighting chance.

If the enamel weakens to the point that it chips off, then a filling needs to be done to remove the affected area and seal it up before it gets worse.

We see a lot of this in our orthodontic braces patients. You see this all the time. The kid goes through braces for a couple of years and when he/she gets their braces off, they have white spots around where the brackets were.

Sometimes these spots are surface spots and can be whitened out. But if he/she didn't brush his/her teeth well during their braces, these defects may be deeper in the enamel. To cover them, bonding or porcelain veneers may be needed.

Along with the decalcification, defective enamel can lead to cold sensitivity because the hard enamel isn't solid anymore and the temperature changes can cause the fluid in the dentin to expand and contract, causing that sharp pain every time you drink/eat something cold.

If I see my orthodontic patients not brushing well, I usually encourage them to use either an over-the-counter Fluoride rinse or a topical toothpaste like MI paste which has extra Fluoride and minerals that will help fight this type of decalcification around the brackets.

As we've talked earlier in the book, decalcification can also be caused by eating/drinking habits such as too much pop or eating a lot of acidic foods like citrus or salsa.

These acidic items can break down the minerals of the enamel faster than the body can heal them and a discolored spot- usually around the gum lines- will appear.

I always encourage my patients to brush very well in these areas and to either use a Fluoride rinse or a topical toothpaste like MI paste to help in these areas so they don't have to come see me for a filling.

Fillings in these areas are not easy for me to place, and they don't tend to last very long because they are thin and tend to be beat up from daily eating.

The last thing your hygienist and or dentist will do is an oral cancer exam. They are generally looking for any bumps, lesions, or areas that are a different color compared to the surrounding tissues.

Let your dentist know if you use any kind of alcohol or tobacco products so he/she can make sure nothing is going on in the mouth!

Chewing tobacco is a whole other story and we can dive into that in the next book, but for now, make sure that your dentist and hygienist know about your usage of these products so they can make sure of early detection!

So listen to the things that are said at your check-up appointment. The hygienist is the first one to see these things and will communicate with the dentist when he/she sees something out of the ordinary.

Ask questions and make sure that you can "get ahead" of these things before they cost you a lot of money as well as a lot of time in the dental chair!

Be proactive in your conversations with your healthcare providers- ask questions- no matter how big or small. Everyone is human! Sometimes things are missed even by the professionals.

But if you notice something with your mouth, or your health in general- get it checked out. With all the advances in modern medicine these days, most things can be reversed, cured, or fixed. But only if you're honest with your healthcare professional and ask questions!

I hope this book answered a lot of questions for you, your friends, and your loved ones. Please share it! If you're in Ohio, come see me- we'd love to see you and help you keep your mouth healthy and strong. If you have any questions, please watch the videos on my website www.akrondentalconcepts.com or email me at docaldrich@gmail.com.

Happy chewing!